Running 101

JEWEL SWEENEY

ISBN:1724637150
ISBN-13:978-1724637154

DEDICATION

To all my people, past and present, who have taken on the challenge of running. You inspired me to put it all on paper and share it with the world.

CONTENTS

ACKNOWLEDGMENTS

Thank you Charlie for spending the late night hours editing and revising with me. And, of course, thank you for taking care of the kids while I write.

Thanks to Anne Samuels for badgering me until I wrote this book.

A thank you to L.C. for dealing with my craziness while trying to put this together and doing the dirty work for me so I could knock this out.

1 INTRODUCTION

I am not a runner. Well, at least not as real runners are concerned. Many people have assumed that I am, but I'm not. Don't get me wrong, I run, but I am not a runner. Runners are a special breed. When you meet a runner, you know.

However, over the last few years, I have become someone who enjoys running. I can say that most days. When I first began running, I had terrible form. The worst part was that I had nobody to tell me. It made me hate running. I ran to lose weight and burn fat. I ran to eat. That was it. My knees would hurt. My lungs would hurt. It was torture. Throughout the last seven years, I have learned a lot about running and have figured out so much that changed my mind on running.

My father was a runner. In high school he set some crazy records for the track team in his main race, the 800 meter. I attended the same high school where his record stood until one of my classmates finally broke it in 2002, 27 years after he set the mark. I am built just like my father, so you would think that I would be able to pick running up and go. I couldn't.

In 2005, during Christmas break, my father and I went for a two mile jog. He smoked me. I mean he embarrassingly crushed me without it being a competition. I was only on break five days because I was on the basketball team for my university. I was in the best shape of my life up until that point. He was gracious and blamed it on my asthma and the cold air.

As much as my lungs did burn from the cold, he beat me because he knew how to run and I didn't. He would give pointers when he could- breathe in and out with your steps, take nice long strides, etc. I used those tips to the best of my ability, but it just didn't click. I was clueless.

It wasn't the last time I would get schooled by an old man running. While preparing for my upcoming wedding day, I attempted to run to lose weight. I was teaching physical education at a high school and had access to the track. I had my planning period first block along with a fellow PE teacher. He was already on the track so I waited for him to pass where I was entering before beginning my run. I thought to myself, "Just stay with him." It wasn't happening. He lapped me. Ugh. Shortly after he passed me, the athletic director came out to ask me a question. He joked about me showing up the older teacher, but I admitted that I had been lapped. Thankfully, he thought I was joking.

So why would I keep going back to running if I was just plain no good at it? Well, for one, I'm competitive. Probably too competitive. So something like running a few miles becomes a challenge I must defeat. The second reason is that I knew what running did for my body. I saw the results of running and, if I could be better at it, I would have a better body. Or at least I hope for that change.

After having my first child I was in desperate need of losing the extra pounds he gave me. In the start of my pursuit to run, I read a book called *Born to Run: A Hidden Tribe, Superathletes, and the Greatest Race the World Has Never Seen* by Christopher McDougall. His words, and findings, changed my life forever. I realized that my "long stride" was way too long. My flouncy running was wasting energy. My tired trodding was destroying my knees. The breathing techniques recommended by my father actually helped me quite a bit, and the focused breathing kept me going, but that was about all I had going for me. Overall, I needed a pretty major reconstruction of my form. *Born to Run* gave me a jump start in the right direction.

Once I applied the techniques discussed in the book, which were minor compared to the actual story that was told, I began to find my stride. I took three minutes off of my 5K time in one run. I was more efficient, and more relaxed. My body took to the adjustments and I had amazing results in my runs and in my weight loss. And, best of all, running became fun.

Now don't get me wrong, it's not like I'm going to go for a run when I just need something to do. But I do enjoy running these days. I enjoy challenging myself to go faster, or to release built up stress. When your body doesn't hurt and you can breathe, running is fun.

I hope that this guide will help anyone who

struggles with running, whether it is a mental struggle or a physical struggle. Through the years I have gained much more knowledge through research, certifications, experience, and training. The goal of this guide is to wrap that knowledge up in a nice neat package without technical jargon using easy to understand language. As fun as it can be to discuss the atrophy of the rectus abdominus and its effects on posture and form, it is better for all to learn in real world terms what can be done to better our runs.

2 REASONS FOR QUITTING

From start to finish, without a doubt, clear as day, the number one reason why people don't keep up with running is their mind. For years I have worked with people who are capable of so much more than they ever attempt. The mind controls the body; the more you believe that, the better you will be, not just at running, but at everything you do.

Often, I see people out of breath as they run. That's great. That's the point of the cardiovascular activity. People often view this strain as a bad thing and go into panic mode. No matter how many times I remind them that there will be a shortness of breath, fear sets in. The fear is the thought that they will run out of air, will pass out, and will end up as road kill.

Understanding that being out of breath in the beginning is natural helps to keep a runner calm. Learning how to control your breathing will change everything. When your mind takes over, your body will follow suit. Your mind might think that the lack of oxygen means you are in distress. It will tell your body to stop putting yourself in this de-oxygenated state. That is, until you take control over your mind.

The mind works off of the nervous system, and fight or flight will set in when under stress.

Those of us that are fighters will enjoy the rush and the battle that happens within us. Those of us that are flight lovers will want to quit immediately because we don't like discomfort in the body.

More than that, our minds have a great deal of pre-existing thoughts about running. Many people begin the process assuming they are going to fail. When I have clients that start off this way I typically will ask, "Then why do you show up to work out? If you think you're going to fail, don't bother. You've made up your mind."

Usually at that point they have decided they should probably start moving. However, the mindset doesn't change to, "Yeah, I can do this." It usually just begins the trail of grumbling. "I hate this. I don't want to do this. Why do we even have to run? My legs hurt. Ugh." Sometimes this grumbling remains only in the mind, other times it spills out into verbal complaints. Depending on the person I will approach this situation in a variety of ways, but the point is always the same-- we were born to run. Our bodies are actually designed for it. There is science to prove it. Running is great for your heart, lungs, bone density, muscles, and hormones. Plus, it is one of the simplest ways to burn fat and get in shape.

The problem is most people just need to get out of their own way. All the negative talk, whether internal or spoken, means the body will follow suit. The mind thinks you are running out of oxygen, so you stop running. The mind says you're too old, too out of shape, too anything, so you stop. Even when you have proper form, there might be times of pain.

Your mind needs to be strong enough to handle running, and the physical challenges that come with it.

I have watched countless people move from "I can't" to "I can't believe it!" And for every one of those, I have watched people with the physical capacity to run better than I ever could just refuse to let their minds run away.

People quit due to mental weakness in many cases. There is always an excuse. There is a stubbornness. There is giant block that stands in their mind that says they just can't run.

If you're reading this handbook, you have figured out that you would like to run, and run well, but you need help. I will tell you this: You need mental fortitude to run on a regular basis. There are going to be hard days. There are going to be long paths and difficult routes. Some days your body will be sore from a previous workout.

You need to enter each run with a plan. Know your route- the miles, the estimated time, the potential hazards or difficult areas, the lighting, the terrain, and anything else. Plan if this is a short, medium, or long run. Set expectations for yourself. Do your best to reach and surpass those expectations. If you don't meet them, don't beat yourself up, just evaluate the run honestly. Was the run harder than expected? Were you more exhausted than you thought you would be? Maybe you just plain had a crummy run. That happens. So you move on to the next one pushing for something better.

The number one reason people quit running

is themselves. Don't let that be you. Be strong. Be prepared.

After the mental challenges that will take place, there are some physical issues that may deter a person from running. Sometimes poor form can lead to nagging pains. They aren't exactly injuries yet, but could be the start of them. Other times people simply feel uncomfortable. Why? It's new! Change bothers many to most humans. We like routines. Our bodies like being at rest. Adding something new, like running, where many people participate and there is a stigma on what people believe runners should look like can be straining on the mind and the body. We must move past it.

Subsequent reasons for quitting would be poor form that leads to injuries and the distaste for running. Both of those can be quenched easily enough. The first solution is just learning proper form, having the right gear, and putting in some slower runs/drill work. The second solution is back to the mental side of running. If you don't like doing it but know you need to give it a fair try, just suck it up and give it a fair try.

3 COMMON RUNNING MISTAKES

There are a variety of mistakes that any one person can make while running. I hope to give you four of the more common mistakes seen in both beginning and regular runners. If we can address these mistakes we can have a relatively quick fix and can keep moving.

The first mistake we will discuss, the shuffle, run is one of the worst mistakes out there. There are a few reasons why one might be shuffling along the streets. When I began running, I was not exactly joyful. After my first run as a mother, my husband asked, "How was the run?" I looked at him with a scowl and said, "That was not a run." He responded with, "Okay, how was the jog?" I was ready to be honest. "It was more like plodding." I was at a partial shuffle stage.

The runner's shuffle is probably the most common form issues I encounter. I see it, and hear it, far too often. The toes scrape into the asphalt and make that grating sound. The shoulders are slumped, the legs are straight, and the runner is often looking like they will fall forward. That shuffle causes both slower times and injuries. Let's look at some of the issues that come from the shuffle and then how we can fix them.

First and foremost we have a slower speed. I don't think I need to unpack this one too much. Any time we have increased friction we will slow down. For those of us trying to speed up our time, we must avoid this shuffling motion. We want to be light on our feet. Picture someone shuffling on the sidewalk. Each step hits with a stopping motion. Obviously, this is the opposite of what we are going for. The friction, the pressure, and the stopping, will all cause a jerking motion. While we run, we want to be smooth.

This shuffling/plodding approach creates heavy feet which can cause injury. It puts a great deal of pressure on the knees in particular. If you watch somebody shuffling down the street you'll see that their legs are often straight when they impact the ground. That means that their knees are absorbing the shock and the weight of their body with each step. Most of us understand that our weight will be absorbed within the joints. The issue we should consider is just how much pressure is coming into these joints. The straighter the leg, the worse the pressure will be.

In addition to all of these joint issues, we have an unusual motion happening with our toes and calves. The foot strike is something we will dive into during our section on form, however we should address it here in the shuffle briefly. Shuffling makes us land on the balls of the feet, or maybe even the toes, causing the calves to work much harder than necessary. Landing on the front of the feet can lead to quicker fatigue of the calf muscles and tendons, and can provoke cramping due to overuse. The bones of the toes are not designed to endure our impact while running, and that impact can produce stress fractures. The shuffle is so common among beginning runners and causes so much damage that hopefully this form can be avoided through education and awareness.

A second mistake, the bounce, is really a simple habit to develop. Many people bounce on the road when running because they began their running journey on a treadmill. Running on a treadmill is a great way to train, particularly in areas where outdoor conditions are poor. But, due to the fear of running off the treadmill or stepping on the front guard, runners will often run up and down, not moving forward. When moving from treadmill to road, I often see that people have kept their treadmill form bouncing up and down. Others bounce simply because they are having so much fun I suppose. I see the flouncy, bouncy air they have and know that they are running for the sake of running. That's all well and good, but that bounce puts increased pressure on the knees and ankles.

A third common sight to see/running mistake is the prance. This occurs when the toe lands with the leg extended. It is more common among young women that are trying to look cute and possibly shed some extra pounds. When the prance is present, there is a good chance that joints are taking impacts that they aren't prepared to take. A great deal of injury can come from the prance because in addition to the length in stride and the straightness of leg, it is near impossible to speed up in this form. This I also know from personal experience. I struggled through the prance for quite some time. It began because I was searching for a longer stride, thinking I would be more efficient. I looked ridiculous. And, I could never speed up my time. It wasn't until I learned to be low and cyclical that I sped up in running.

This next mistake, our fourth to discuss, is an easy one to spot but sometimes the most difficult to fix. The speed walk jog is more common with people starting in their 40's or older. Sometimes younger people will develop this habit when they join their parents on runs or begin their journey as severely obese individuals. Too often people begin jogging by simply speeding up their walk, which looks almost like the prance, but many times it can be a slow, very slow, run.

There are two reasons for why someone may be doing the speed walk jog. The first, as mentioned previously, is from physical obesity. But even that falls under a larger umbrella – fear, which is reason number two. Being overweight, having knee injuries, or other issues, can cause a fear that makes one timid in the art of running. It's as if the brain says, "I know my body will hold me when I walk, but the pressure from running will make my legs snap to pieces!" And so the runner takes these light and easy speed walker steps. I often see this style with my clients. They know they must perform some variation of running, but are quite unsure of themselves and their body so they gently speed up from a walk. It doesn't fool me but, as their trainer, I need to battle their minds if I'm going to get them to run correctly. Fear needs to be eliminated.

4 COMMON INJURIES

When it comes to running there are a variety of injuries that are possible. The goal of this booklet is not to help you self diagnose, but to get you to understand what might be happening to your body when you feel something that makes you say, "Ow." As many of you might already know, the majority of injuries will be in the lower body. However, there are a few upper body issues that may have to get worked on as well.

Let's begin with what might be the most common injury, shin splints. I was taking a course on Running Injury Prevention several years ago and the writer of the manual was discussing shin splints and said, "…we still don't know the cause of shin splints…". That point convinced me that I might know more than I thought. We do know the cause of shin splints. Let me try to break it down into common terminology. Your bones are covered in what is called the periosteum. It's like a sleeve. When you run or jump and increase the use of the muscles around the lower leg (the soleus; the gastrocnemius; and the anterior tibialis) the muscles contract and release. If those muscles are over-contracting, it pulls on the periosteum. Easily stated, the muscles pull the sleeve and it hurts.

This over-contraction can be from a variety of issues, some of which I will try to cover here. The easiest way that people will try to fix shin splints is to exercise on a more buoyant surface. If you're running on cement (like sidewalks), it has no give. It will create more force on the joints and the muscles will work harder to absorb that additional force.

If the shin splints are bad enough, you will need to rest, ice, and take anti-inflammatory medicines. Once you are taken care of, evaluate the surface you are running on. The first option is to move to asphalt or even grass to run. Typically that will help. It could also be a quick fix with shoes. The heel may be too large, the arches could be too high or too low. These are simple fixes that should be checked first.

Sometimes the issue is slightly more difficult. When form is involved, it can take longer to figure out and then fix. The most common issue I see is that people are running with their toes lifted too high. To raise the toes, you must engage the anterior tibialis. So, if you have gone from walking to trying your hand (or feet!), at running, you are likely to raise your toe to get your foot to your next step. To fix that motion, you must raise the knee and relax the foot more. Again, more difficult to fix than changing where you run or buying some new shoes.

Another common injury that is related to shin splints is plantar fasciitis. This injury is also caused by overuse. The continual pounding on the foot can be caused by the terrain, shoes, or poor form.

Plantar fasciitis is pretty easy to diagnose. It is often described as if you are walking on rocks. There is inflammation and pain through the fascia . (that is basically the bottom) of the foot. The inflammation and pain can vary from person to person, but the overall consensus is that it is a quite painful. Part of the issue of the pain is that if you are an active person, or just on your feet enough at work, there is very little rest time for the injury to heal and your body recover.

The best treatment for this injury is rest. The miles added through running will aggravate the injury and thus it will take longer to heal. When resting, ice will help to bring down the inflammation. I was once told that a frozen water bottle is a great way to reduce the swelling. It was great advice. During my personal battle, I used the frozen water bottle by placing it on the floor and rolling the foot back and forth on it. It will start off painful, but the sooner you start, the better. There is also a "night brace" you can purchase that will stretch your foot. It is recommended that you wear it for eight hours, so most people wear it at night while they're sleeping.

A third obstacle, muscle cramps, are quite common in all fitness, but especially in running. All cramps occur for the same reason – a lack of oxygen. When there isn't enough oxygen in blood cells, the cells create a cramping effect in the muscles. For instance, people that haven't learned how to breathe well when running, may not have taken in enough oxygen through their breaths. That creates the age old stitch in the side. The way to get through it? Deep breathing.

Cramps in muscles have plagued runners since we began the jogging phase. Our bodies excrete "trash" on a cellular level. Simplest way to explain it is this: the cells use the oxygen and exchange it with trash. The trash gets left in the blood stream. An unequal balance of trash and oxygen creates a cramp. To release the cramp there are a variety of options. During the cramp, say a charley horse, place one hand on either side of the muscle and help the muscle contract. When you help the muscles contract, it quickens the pace with which the muscle gets to fatigue. From there, the muscle will be too tired to contract and you will get some peace. This is the concept behind e-stim or electrical stimulation. The shocks of the machine force the muscle to contract and essentially tire it out. That, however, is not an avenue that many people have on hand but you may experience it in a rehab facility or someplace similar.

So what about the trash? Well, drinking water will help. Sports drinks can also help clear the blood stream of junk. However, the top dog of relieving cramps is actually chocolate milk. The research is over a decade old, and still holds true. The main item of trash is lactic acid. That acidity in the muscle is what causes the pain and cramp. So, the lactose of the chocolate milk clears that out from the system. Why the chocolate? The sugar. It gets the lactose into the blood stream faster. So hopefully you aren't lactose intolerant. I've had many clients that turn their nose up to milk and chocolate milk. From personal experience, I can say that feel sorry for them. I have had such great relief from it. Plus, I love the taste!

A final common injury that I will discuss is simple muscle soreness. It is typically assumed that our legs will be sore from the running. Anytime we add new exercises we will have soreness. When we add weight bearing exercises, that soreness increases. Unfortunately, there isn't too much we can do for soreness. We must warm up the muscles properly using dynamic stretches. It is important that our muscles are warm and ready for running, but are not overly stretched (yes, that's a thing!). After running, it is a good idea to do your static stretches. Foam rollers are good for both pre- and post- workout muscle release.

What might surprise runners are the pains and aches of muscles and joints outside of the legs. Often, when I see runners attempting to speed up, they tense up. When that happens, the shoulders usually shrug up towards the ears. The complaint will be a tightness and stiffness in the neck and upper trapezius muscles. To combat this, there will need to be a conscious effort of relaxing the upper body while running. We can sometimes use our breathing to help relax the shoulders and neck.

The back can be another troublesome area. If you are running with proper form, the hamstrings will be used more often than the quadriceps. When the hamstrings take on a greater workload, flexibility is extremely important. Tight hamstrings can cause problems with the knees and, more often, the back. The old song discussing how everything is connected has some validity to it. The hamstrings attach higher than most people realize into the hip girdle and as the muscles pull the hip girdle they can affect the tilt of the hips and then pull against the back muscles. Again, we can turn to flexibility and proper stretching (before and after) to relieve our aches and soreness. The piriformis stretch is a great addition to any routine, but especially if you have tight hamstrings and experience back pain.

5 FORM

We've looked at the reasons people quit, some mistakes they make, and some common injuries. Now let's take a look at the very thing that can clear up all three of those concerns- our form. Many people think that the thing to do is just go out and see what happens. That isn't exactly a terrible idea. One way that I teach people that are struggling to find proper form is to play a game of tag or to chase their dog around the back yard. The brain often interferes with running. It continues to give us directions on what to do and how to do it, so much so that we can't think clearly. We tense up, our breathing gets in the way, and we finally are just in too much pain to do anything. Worst of all, you probably did worse than if you had just let go and run around.

So if you have been running around but you're plagued with injuries, mishaps, or maybe something doesn't feel right, let's get down to the form we should have. We will look at posture, stride, and foot strike. Each of these work together to help you get where you need to go.

Before we get into the big three items, I would like to provide a reminder about muscle usage. We will talk both about distance running and sprints. When running distance, there is a more relaxed feel and the legs should be pushing with the hamstrings as the primary mover. Sprinting requires everything to be tight and in place. Every joint has a job. When you sprint, the quadriceps are in charge of pulling the knee up in a driving motion. As we look at our form, keep this information in mind as you are picturing yourself running, and then as you are performing the runs desired.

Posture is a simple fix for most, but can be tricky for those that run post lifting or during times of fatigue in general. Distance running requires a straight back with your shoulders up. American culture has allowed slouching all too often. When we have a straight back and our shoulders up and back, we can keep our heads up. Many people want to look at the ground a step or two ahead of themselves. This motion is quite detrimental to your form and to your body as a whole. The chin being up will allow the shoulders to be located over the hips. When the shoulders slump and we are looking down, we end up leaning forward ever so slightly. For some people, the lean is greater and will cause even more damage. Leaning over will not allow for your hamstrings to push your knees forward enough. It will bring about the shuffle or a pounding. The knees will absorb the weight of the runner as they hit the ground. Each step becomes more of a jolt than it should be. With your shoulders and head up, the legs can be pushed out in front of you.

One way to get your legs out and moving in the right direction is to lower the hips. I know that this sounds awkward, but after you put it into practice it will feel better. As a basketball player I was taught to sit in my shot, meaning to catch the ball with your booty dropping to a squat or half squat so that you can explode- be it jumping up to shoot, or taking off dribbling. So I understand the concept a little further than most. When we are in a lowered position, our legs are given more options for movement. It also stabilizes the core and upper body. Being steady and having minimal upper body movement helps keep the motion in the legs. The shoulders will roll naturally with our steps, but our arms should be relaxed. Distance running needs to be comfortable.

The posture for sprinting is entirely different. We want that lean over. The difference is that it is purposeful. Sprinters do not lean and bend at the waist. There is, essentially, a straight line from the shoulders to the heels. To accomplish this form, the lean is more like letting gravity drag you down. The angle of which Olympic sprinters run, off the blocks, is 30°. That is a ridiculous angle to attain as an amateur runner. There are ways to practice this, typically in partnership. However, if you are on your own and have the opportunity of a straight lane without traffic, you can practice leaning in sprinting. While leaning the shoulders forward, drive the knees to the chest. This will lengthen the stride. It will be a challenge, but press the hips forward to create a straight line with your body. When you feel like you're falling and simply catching yourself repeatedly, that is a good sign. You are on your way to great sprinting. It will take baby steps, but that is where you start.

As for arms while sprinting, we have a much different process from distance running. The elbows should be bent at ninety degrees. While taking an outstanding track and field class at Charleston Southern University, the track coach was our professor. He had a no nonsense approach to class and I could see why he had such a winning record as coach. He told us our hands needed to go "cheek to cheek." What that breaks down to is that as your arms are at ninety degrees, you drive your elbows up and back. One hand should reach your cheek on your face while the other hand has reached the cheek of your, well, you know what. The driving force of the elbows working with the driving force of the knees will keep your body moving forward and staying balanced. Your hands should be open and straight.

The next issue is our stride. As a beginner, I was told to have a long stride. The problem was that I let my previous ballet experience take over and I felt like a gazelle. I might have looked like one too. A busted up gazelle, at least. When I was first taught to have a long stride, I wasn't told to keep my posture tight. So there I was thinking that I needed to keep going longer. My legs straightened. Our stride needs to be more rounded than I ever expected. Going through trainings and reading, I learned that many professional runners use biking as a major training technique because it maintains their form while keeping them from weight bearing activities.

A rounded stride is the clear way to go. We

do many drills, whether as a warm up or for cardiovascular health, that are actually the breakdowns of proper form. Doing high knees and butt kicks are familiar exercises for any former athlete. Doing high knees with purpose, sometimes slower even, will help develop the form to use the knees coming up. When the knees come up, it allows for the foot to fall easily to the ground. The motion of the butt kick brings the heel up and the knee back a bit. So now we combine the two-- the heel coming back allows the knee to drive forward into the form of the high knee and we place the foot down with ease and kick it back again.

As for the length of the stride, you'll notice that your legs will reach farther when your posture is better. If your shoulders round, your knee will not be able to come forward as easily. Small strides are a sign of the knees not moving up and out. You'll find a stride length that feels comfortable for you. When that happens, enjoy it. If there is pain, you'll need to adjust. Finding the right stride may take time, but as you run it will click.

Foot strike is connected greatly to the stride. If the stride is too long, you'll most likely be running heel to toe. When the foot strike is too short, there will be a lot of shuffling. Personally, I like to listen to the first strike before I watch it. Running shouldn't sound like the herd of elephants got released from the zoo. We're bound to hear our steps, but they should be light and soft. Believe it or not, the science of exercise physiology has actually figured out that a mid-foot strike is the best placement to run on.

That "ball of the foot" always seemed a little awkward, right? It has all this added cushion. Why? So we too can bounce a little. It allows for a little give as we land. The arch of the foot can be strange as well. It acts like a rubber band and stretches out as you land and retracts when you are off of it. So when we run and land on our toes, the absorption of force goes into our knees. When we land on our heels the absorption goes to the heel and ankle. Think of your body as a glass vase wrapped for moving. You put plenty of bubble wrap around the bottom, but forget to double up as the vase goes higher. As long as the vase is placed so the bottom absorbs the bumps on the ride, you're okay! If the vase gets hit from the sides, you're likely to smash it to pieces. The bottom of our foot has bubble wrap in the ball of the foot and the arch. When we hit the mid-foot strike, we all for the bubble wrap to do its job.

How do we ensure that mid-foot strike? Using proper form, like a higher knee, allows the foot to come down where it needs to. If our foot kicks out further than our knee, our heel will hit first. If our legs are too straight we will hit toe first. The rounded stride will allow for a mid-foot strike. And, of course, the rounded stride is made possible by proper posture.

6 BREATHING

Now that we have our form in place we can talk about breathing throughout our run. B-reathe it or not, this is important. As I mentioned in the introduction, my father was a huge help in getting me to breathe well enough to get the running in. He taught me to breathe with my steps. "In two, three, four. Out two, three, four." Some people choose to breathe with a three beat when they begin this method. Many people suggest that we breathe in through the nose and out through the mouth. This method also keeps our breathing steady as we exercise.

One of the biggest issues I come across is panicked breathing. In this scenario, what happens is more mental than physical. However, the mental side will tell the physical side just what to do. Many people become so anxious over the thought of running – possible injuries, losing their breath and passing out, pain, cramps, you name it – that they put themselves into a minor panic attack. Breathing becomes rapid and shallow, and they've only run a few steps. This is dangerous for a variety of reasons. First, naturally, the body will feel the effects of shallow, rapid breathing by becoming dizzy and weak. Second, the mind will store running as a negative thing. Third, the panicked breathing will continue through every run you attempt to take because of this single event.

Let's combat the panic with a sense of calm. Now I'm not up to snuff on all my mind and body lingo, so let's just start here. Before you begin your run, take a deep breath in, hold it a bit, and release it calming your body and mind. Fix your eyes on a target ahead of you and know that it will all be alright. Nobody expects to see you battling for the title at the next Boston Marathon (but if you are, let me know because I'll watch!) Take a second deep breath and begin running. Keep a steady rhythm in your head to breathe in and out, whether with your steps or a mantra you make for yourself. I like to repeat, "Light, easy, smooth," to the steps. Light refers to the sound of my steps. Easy refers to my breathing. And smooth is how I should look to others.

The "easy" referenced above is something that can cause some difficulty and confusion for some. Technically, "easy" means that we are not running in such a way that a strain could hinder us. Actually, there shouldn't be any strain when we are running. The confusion comes to people both athletic and non-athletic. For the athlete mentality, people often struggle with the idea that anything should be easy. Easy equals no to little results. For the non-athlete, easy means we should never have a hard run. Truth is, there needs to be a middle ground to this mentality.

In order to find out how strenuous an exercise or a workout is, personal trainers have learned to use the talk test with their clients. The talk test is where the trainer will ask the client to recite the Pledge of Allegiance or sing the ABC's, or something similar that they would know. Once they are speaking, we judge the breathing capacity. If the participant in the activity can speak or sing without any problems, than the exercise exertion was not at max capacity. We call this the VO2max or threshold. Basically, the goal is to find exactly when you are out of breath. When we fall under that VO2max, we are capable of more. Now, whether or not that feels easy to you is really at your discretion. Athletes that are used to reaching their VO2max during competition will often run at the peak of this threshold. It may be a strain, but the challenge is what most athletes enjoy.

For someone just starting out, the VO2max will probably be much lower than athletes, but there will still be one. The goal is to run under that max, but not too far below. When I perform that test with my clients and they go through the Pledge of Allegiance without so much as a single pause to breathe, I point out that they might not be working hard enough. Finding that balance takes practice without someone over your shoulder. And for most people starting without athletic backgrounds, and even some with, it can be difficult to find that sweet spot.

Breathing for sprinting is entirely different. Sprints are anaerobic. I'm sure we all know what they mean, but just in case – Aerobic means with oxygen, anaerobic means without oxygen. That is the most basic way to explain it, though science provides us with some deeper processes happening within the body. So basically what we need to know is that distance running should be continual deeper breaths, while sprinting is short distances and uses less oxygen.

In high school I was trained, and I use the word lightly, as a sprinter. To me, breathing for sprints feels like a 90's sitcom version of lamaze classes. He-hoo-he-hoo-he-hoo. Now, we still want those deep breaths as much as possible, but our bodies are moving too fast for them. I tried to focus on breathing recently during my last few sprints and it holds true what I learned in high school. The emphasis is more on the exhale than the inhale. We've witnessed this in weight training. The big exhale (sometimes a grunt, growl, or yell) when the big push comes. Similarly, sprinting is all a big push. From the angle to the physiology, it is all about power. Those breaths will help to give that power.

7 SPEEDING UP

Speeding up goes hand in hand with breathing, at least from what I have found to work. Many of my clients have started running and begin with a nice slow and steady mentality. The fear of being out of breath keeps runners at a slower pace as we discussed earlier. So when the time comes to get that pace time in a happier zone, how do we do that?

First, we have to get over the fact that we will in fact breathe harder. Our legs will hurt a little more. If we want new results, we will have to do something new. And that means we will be uncomfortable.

The method that I have found to work well is to time my breathing with my increasing speed. The first part of it is just like beginning to run, taking a deep breath in mid stride. As you exhale, speed up a bit. Stick with that speed for as long as you can. If you feel you can speed up again, proceed in the same manner. During this time of finding a new speed, you many notice that you are inconsistent. You speed up and slow down. The ultimate goal is to get faster little by little.

The deep exhale technique works for me because I am able to then reset my breathing to match my steps as they speed up. It gives me a good four count to get my legs moving faster and begin breathing properly. I notice within this technique that I may slow down a good bit after a few minutes of the faster pace. For some people that change in pace is a huge hindrance because we have worked so hard feeling the intensity in our steps, but our overall time doesn't change. I force myself on my shorter runs to truly push myself and, when I feel the slow down happening, I need to immediately recognize it and go back to the faster pace.

When you choose to speed up, you may want to start with shorter distances. If your longest runs are 3 miles or so, you might start the speeding up process with fartleks. Fartleks are a Swedish training that has been used for multiple decades all around the world. The basic description is that you sprint for a set distance or time, then jog or walk for a designated distance or time. This repetition of sprinting builds your VO2max. This will make it easier as you run distance runs to speed up and to breathe deeper.

Another option for increasing your speed is to choose a short distance like a mile, or maybe just a half mile, and run as fast as you can without it turning into a sprint. Remember, sprinting is a whole different game. The form changes, the breathing changes. It's anaerobic exercise. So we want to run a shorter distance at a faster pace while still using oxygen. It's tricky, but it certainly works. As your runs grow in distance and time, the short runs should also increase, that is when we will see the differences between a fast run and a sprint.

The last method I will give you to speed up is the treadmill. For some of you, the music began playing and you started dancing. "Finally! Treadmill!" I believe that most of us though, we heard a dirge. When using a treadmill you can choose your speed. Obviously, if we have a treadmill making us run faster, we will! Or maybe you'll choose to fall and become a viral video or simply step off the machine. The point is that we have an outside control mechanism that will get you to train at a faster speed. Although these points can be used in a 5k or a 10k, we want to incorporate them into our regular training routines.

Remember that mantra we stole from *Born to Run*? "Light, easy, smooth," are three words that can take you a long way. Smooth was always something I was trying to attain. Booty down, little work in the upper body, and all those things we have been working on, were what I thought would lead me to being smooth as I ran. I continually show myself it is most often when I am working on speeding up my pace that I am smoother than I was. The legs know what to do. When you shut your brain up, take a deep breath, and run, your body will go and the legs can take you through. The next thing you know, your eyes are fixed on a sign a quarter mile away and you realize you aren't bouncing like you used to. So when you speed up, work to get yourself to smooth and you'll see great results.

8 ADDING MILES

If we've reached this point, we know how to run. We are getting faster each month. But now we're getting a little bored, maybe a little too comfortable. What do we do now? It might be time to log more miles to create a new challenge. Perhaps you bought this whole booklet because you want to run a half marathon or a marathon and you thought, "I just need to add miles." Okay, probably not that last one. Now is the time of the journey we make things a little more interesting.

For many people, adding miles isn't high on the list of things to do. For many, just attempting to run and getting in two miles is more than enough. However, we need to cover how to add miles because we all can't just run a half mile and call it quits. Everyone at one point or another will need this secret recipe for continued results. And I do mean secret.

Just a few years ago, a client had told me how badly she wanted to run six miles. It was a dream to her. I asked how far she was running now and she said three, sometimes three and a half miles. "How will I be able to do it?" she begged me. I got real quiet because I knew people around were listening on the edge of their seat. "Just go do it," I told her plainly. I'm telling you, Nike got it right. If you want something, you need to go out there and do it. The only person stopping you from running further is you. Fear kicks in, we think our bodies can't handle it or we will run out of oxygen, as if there is a shortage somewhere.

You may need to slow your pace back down, maybe for a few miles to get the distance you want. The thing to do is focus on your goal. If the goal is to add miles, just do it. Whether it is at a slow pace, or a fast pace, or a pace in between, doesn't matter. Run the miles. It is the simplest part of all of running. There will be hesitation and second guessing, but the thrill you receive after finishing a longer run will keep you hooked. You'll have more and more challenges as time goes on, but they will be challenges we want to face and overcome.

9 A FINAL WORD

Running can be a lot of fun when done with proper form and technique. The last thing you want is to be plagued with injuries and struggles. Whether you are running for fun, for exercise, or for competition, there is always a reason to run. I hope that this booklet helped you to figure out some of the issues you may have been having or perhaps has given you the confidence to step out and lace up those shoes.

Throughout it all, we must keep in mind that there will be good days and bad. The goal is to simply have more good days than the bad ones. One thing to keep in mind to have these good days is that you must cross train. No great athlete becomes the best by only pursuing that one part of their training. You must add strength training. There should be a variety of cardiovascular activities as well, both weight bearing and non. Keep in mind all the muscles that are working, and that each of those muscle groups will need a break.

If you are looking for specific workouts with days, distances, and times, I encourage you to seek a professional. There are many workouts online available to you. Some will be tremendous, others not so much. Do your research. Find someone with credentials to get you where you want to be.

    Thank you all for joining me on our trek through Running 101. Happy Running!

ABOUT THE AUTHOR

Jewel Sweeney is a wife and mother of two living in South Carolina. She is the author of a variety of books, fiction and non-fiction alike. Jewel is a Certified Personal Trainer through the American Council on Exercise (ACE). She holds specialist certifications in Running Injury Prevention, Triathlon Injury Prevention, Fitness Nutrition for Sport and Health, and Weight Loss Management.

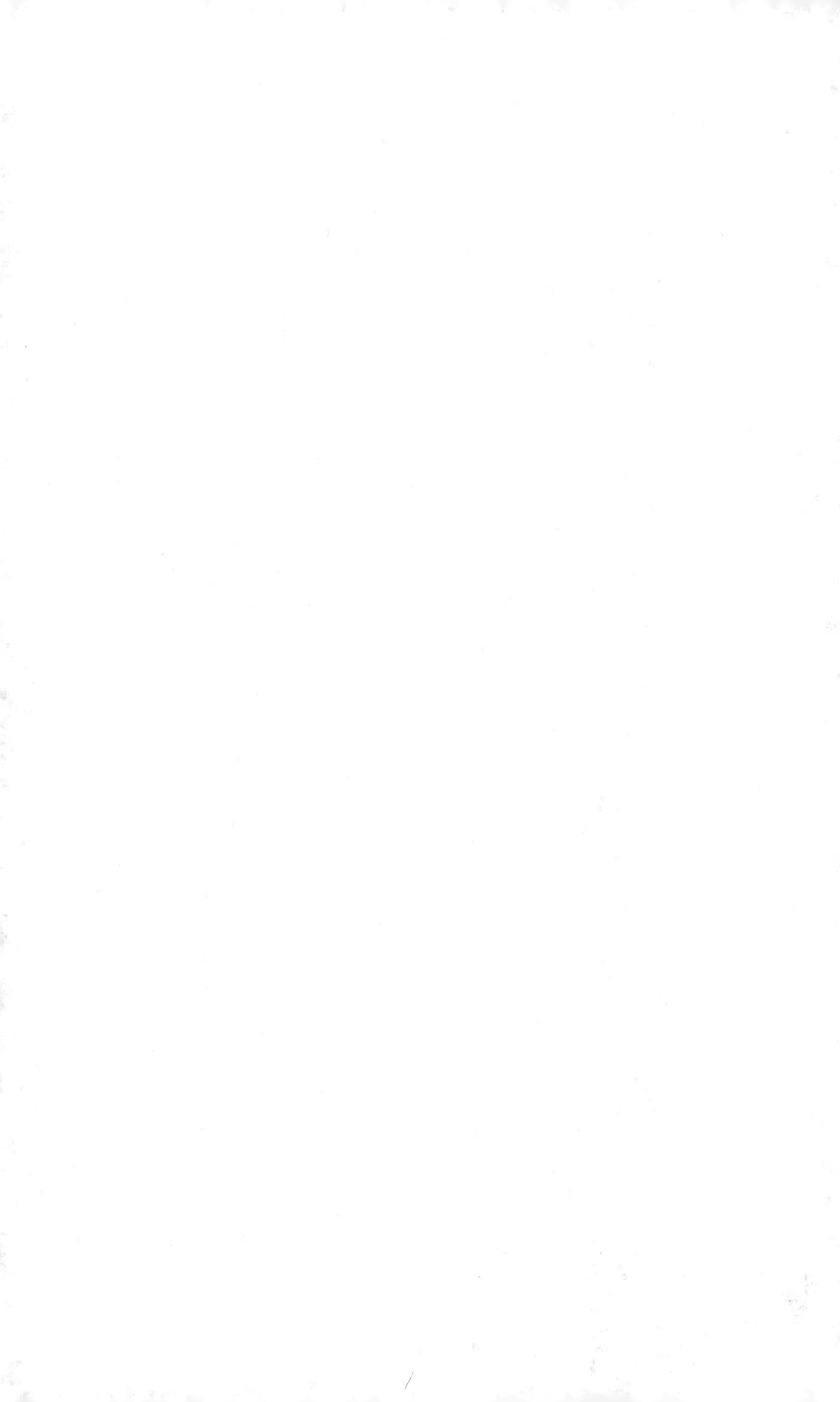